# The Super Easy Plant-Based Recipe Book

Quick and Cheap Plant-Based Recipes to Improve Your Diet and Boost Your Meals

Clay Palmer

# Table of Contents

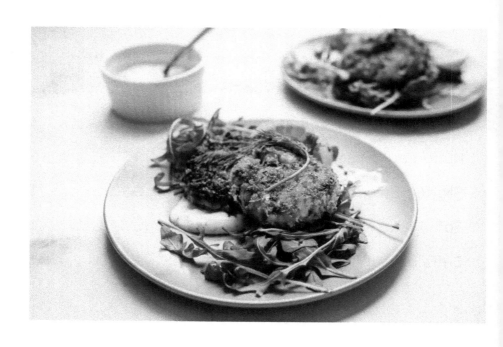

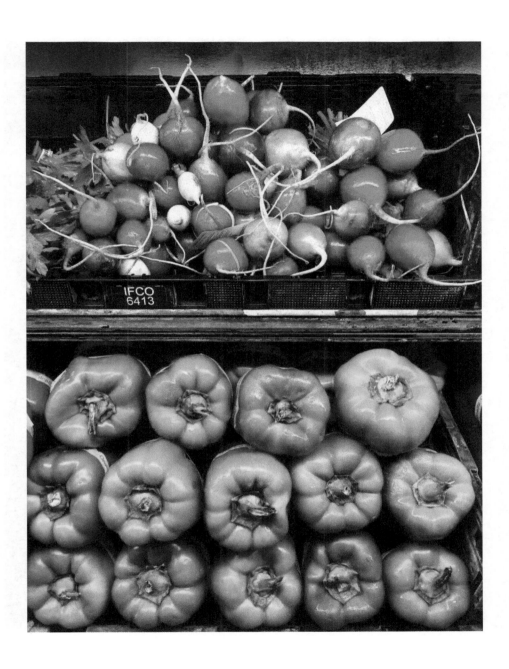

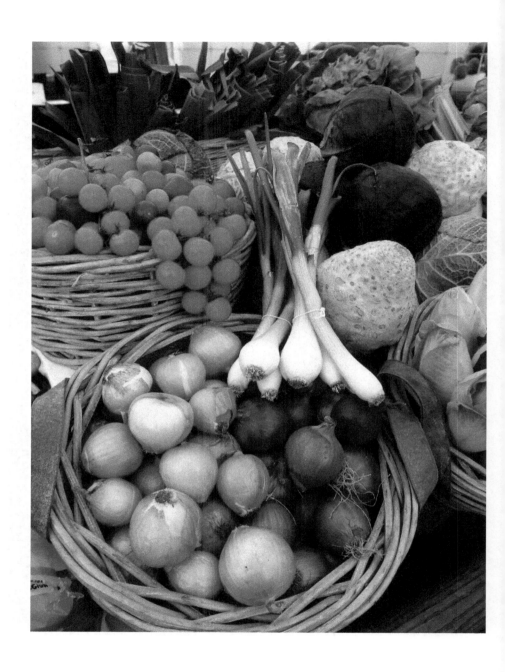

## Pumpkin Penne

Preparation time: 10 minutes

Cooking time: 60 minutes

Servings: 4

### Ingredients:

½ of medium white onion, sliced into wedges 2 cloves of garlic, unpeeled 1 cup cooked and mashed sugar pie pumpkin ½ cup unsalted cashews, soaked, drained ½ teaspoon of sea salt 1/3 teaspoon ground black pepper 5 fresh sage leaves 2 tablespoons olive oil and more as needed for drizzling 1 cup vegetable broth 16 ounces penne pasta, cooked

**Directions:** Take a baking sheet, place onion, pumpkin and garlic in it, drizzle with salt, season with salt and black pepper, pierce pumpkin with a fork, cover the baking sheet and bake for 45 minutes until vegetables are very tender. Then add sage in the last five minutes and after 45 minutes of baking, uncover the baking sheet and continue baking for 15 minutes. When done, peel the pumpkin add to the food processor along with remaining vegetables and ingredients, except for pasta and puree until blended. Place pasta in a pot, add half of the blended pumpkin mixture, stir until coated, then stir in remaining pumpkin mixture and serve.

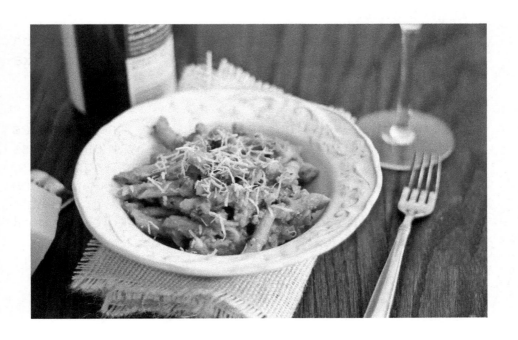

## Sweet Potato Fries

Preparation time: 10 minutes

Cooking time: 30 minutes

Servings: 4

### Ingredients:

3 large sweet potatoes 1/2 teaspoon sea salt ¼ teaspoon cayenne pepper 1 teaspoon cumin 1/4 teaspoon paprika 1 tablespoon olive oil

**Directions:** Peel the potatoes, cut into wedges lengthwise, place them in a bowl, drizzle with oil and toss until combined. Stir together remaining ingredients, sprinkle over sweet potatoes, spread the potatoes evenly on a baking sheet greased with oil in a single layer, and bake for 30 minutes at 400 degrees F until done, tossing twice. Serve straight away.

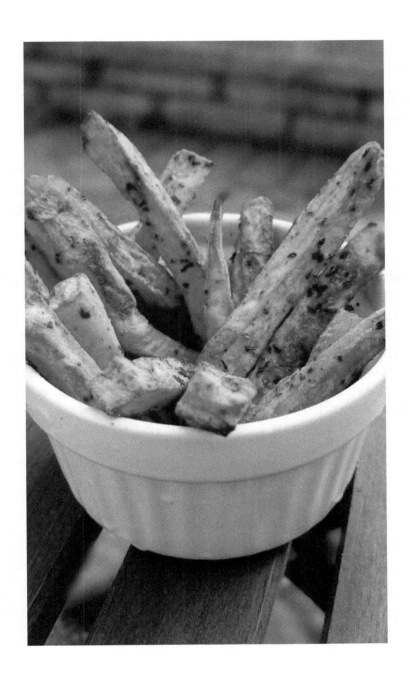

## Roasted Cauliflower

Preparation time: 10 minutes

Cooking time: 1 hour and 20 minutes

Servings: 4

**Ingredients:** 1 medium head of cauliflower ½ teaspoon salt 1 teaspoon dried parsley 1 teaspoon dried dill 1 teaspoon dried mint 1 tablespoon zaatar spice 2 tablespoons olive oil, divided 1 cup of water

**Directions:** Trim the cauliflower, then slice from the bottom, drizzle it with 1 tablespoon oil, season with salt and zaatar spice, cover cauliflower with a foil and bake for 55 minutes. When done, uncover the cauliflower, drizzle with remaining oil and bake for 30 minutes until roasted, turning halfway. When done, sprinkle with parsley, dill, and milk and serve cauliflower with lemon wedges and tahini sauce.

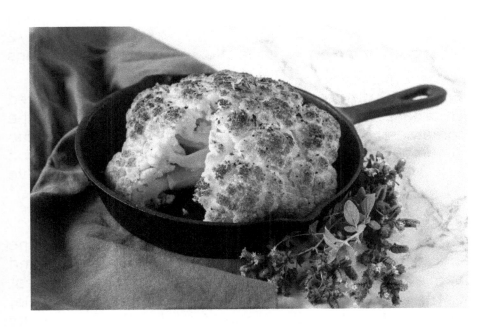

## Quinoa Cakes

Preparation time: 20 minutes

Cooking time: 25 minutes

Servings: 4

### Ingredients:

**For the Quinoa Cakes:** 1 cup quinoa, rinsed 1 teaspoon garlic powder 1/2 teaspoon salt 1 teaspoon cumin 1/2 teaspoon Italian dried herbs 1 lemon, zested 2 teaspoons olive oil 2 cups of water 1/4 cup chopped parsley

**For the Tomato Chickpea Relish** 1 ½ cup cooked chickpeas 1/4 cup chopped scallions 2 cups grape tomatoes, halved 1/4 cup chopped fresh basil 1 cup cucumber, diced ¼ teaspoon minced garlic 1/4 teaspoon salt 3 tablespoons balsamic vinegar 3 tablespoons olive oil

**Directions:** Take a pot over high heat, add all the ingredients for quinoa in it except for lime zest and parsley, stir, bring the mixture to boil, then switch heat to the low level and simmer for 20 minutes. Meanwhile, prepare tomato relish and for this, place all its ingredients in a bowl and stir until combined. When quinoa has cooked, let it stand for 5 minutes, then fluff it with a fork, cool it for 15 minutes, stir in parsley and lemon zest and shape the mixture into four balls. Fry the balls over medium heat on a greased pan for 5 minutes until browned, then transfer them on a plate, top with chickpea relish and serve.

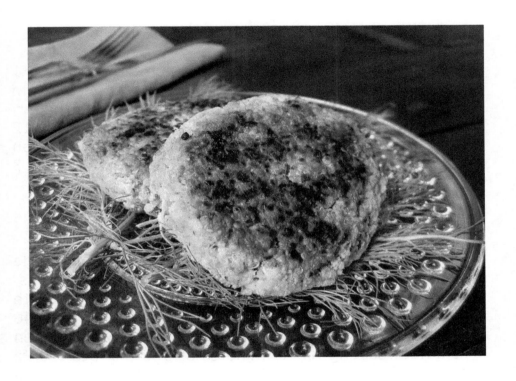

# Ratatouille

Preparation time: 5 minutes

Cooking time: 15 minutes

Servings: 4

## Ingredients:

2 medium zucchini, sliced into ½-inch sliced moons 1 large eggplant, cut into ½-inch pieces 2 medium tomatoes, cut into ¾-inch wedges 1 red bell pepper, sliced into ½-inch strips 1 medium white onion, sliced 12 cloves of garlic, peeled 1 teaspoon salt 1 teaspoon balsamic vinegar 1/3 teaspoon ground black pepper 3 tablespoons rosemary and thyme Olive oil as needed

## Directions:

Prepare all the vegetables, then spread them in a single layer on a greased sheet pan, add garlic and herbs, drizzle with oil, toss until coated and season with salt with black pepper. Toss the vegetables, roast them for 40 minutes at 400 degrees F, tossing halfway, and then continue roasting for 20 minutes at 300 degrees F until tender. When done, taste to adjust salt, drizzle with vinegar and serve.

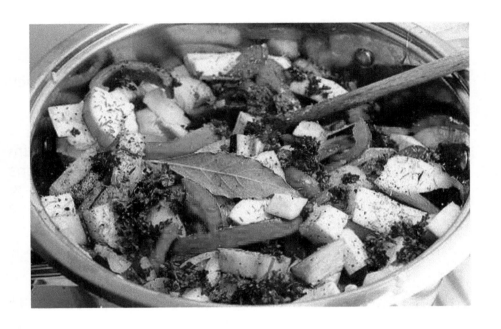

## Blackened Tempeh

Preparation time: 10 minutes

Cooking time: 10 minutes

Servings: 2

### Ingredients:

### For the Ranch Dressing:

1 teaspoon Cajun spice blend 1/3 cup vegan ranch dressing

### For the Blackened Tempeh:

4 radishes, sliced 3 cups shredded kale 1 medium avocado, pitted, sliced 1 block of tempeh 3 tablespoons Cajun Spice ½ a lemon, zested ¼ cup pickled onions ¼ teaspoon salt 1 teaspoon peanut oil 2 tablespoons olive oil 1 scallion, sliced

### Directions:

Prepare the ranch dressing and for this, place all its ingredients in a bowl and stir until combined, set aside until required. Take a sauté pan, place it over medium heat, add tempeh, pour in salted water to cover it, and simmer for 8 minutes until its bitterness has reduced. When done, transfer tempeh to a cutting board, then cut it ½-inch slices and season with Cajun spices until coated on both sides. Place shredded kale in a bowl, drizzle with peanut oil, season with salt and lemon zest, massage with fingers, then add remaining ingredients along with ranch dressing and toss until coated. Distribute the kale salad between the bowl, top with tempeh and scallions and then serve.

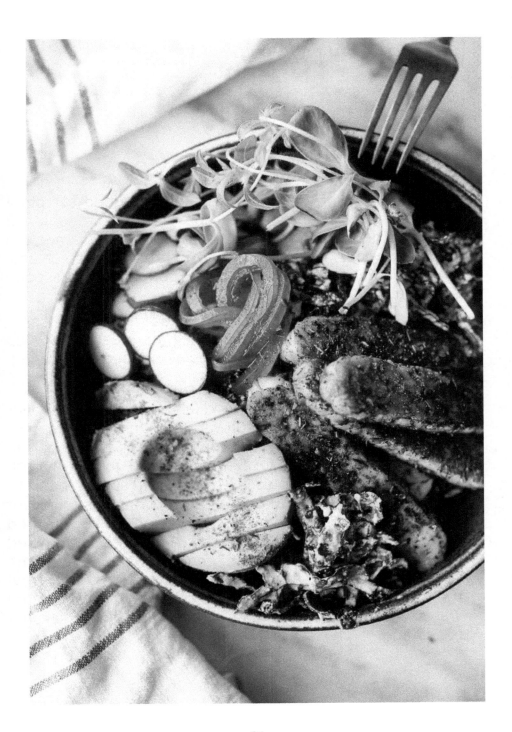

## Szechuan Tofu and Veggies

Preparation time: 10 minutes

Cooking time: 20 minutes

Servings: 2

### Ingredients:

8 ounces tofu, drained, cubed 1 cup shredded carrots 4 ounces sliced mushrooms ½ cup sliced white onion 2 cups shredded cabbage 1 cup asparagus ½ of medium red bell pepper, cored, sliced 8 dried red Chinese chilies, small 1/3 teaspoon ground black pepper 2/3 teaspoon salt 2 tablespoons olive oil

**For Garnish:** Chopped scallions as needed Sesame seeds as needed Red chili flakes as needed ¼ cup Szechuan Sauce Zucchini noodles as needed for serving

**Directions:** Take a large skillet pan, place it over medium heat, add oil, season with salt and black pepper, then season tofu with ½ teaspoon, add it to the pan in an even layer and cook for 5 minutes until golden on both sides. Transfer tofu pieces to a plate, switch heat to medium-high level, add onion and mushrooms, cook for 3 minutes, then switch heat to medium level, add remaining vegetables along with chilies, toss until mixed and cook for 5 minutes until tender-crisp. Pour in the sauce, toss until coated, cook for 2 minutes, then add tofu pieces, stir until coated, and cook for 2 minutes until warm. When done, sprinkle with scallions and sesame seeds and serve over zucchini noodles.

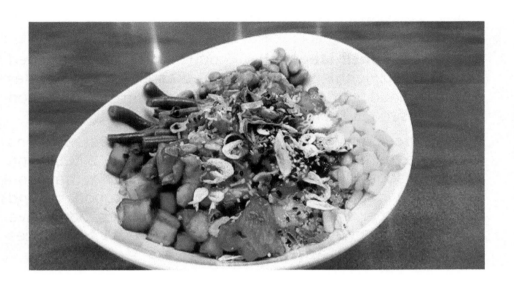

# Lentil Meatballs with Coconut Curry Sauce

Preparation time: 15 minutes

Cooking time: 60 minutes

Servings: 14

## Ingredients:

**For the Lentil Meatballs:** 6 ounces tofu, firm, drained 1 cup black lentils ½ cup quinoa 1 teaspoon garlic powder 1 teaspoon salt 1/3 cup chopped cilantro 1 teaspoon fennel seed 1 Tablespoon olive oil

**For the Curry:** 1 large tomato, diced 2 teaspoons minced garlic 1 tablespoon grated ginger 1 teaspoon brown sugar ½ teaspoon ground turmeric ¼ teaspoon cayenne pepper ½ teaspoon salt ¼ teaspoon ground black pepper 1 tablespoon lime juice 2 tablespoons olive oil 1 tablespoon dried fenugreek leaves 13.5 ounces coconut milk, unsweetened

## Directions:

 Boil lentils and fennel in 3 cups water over high heat, then simmer for 25 minutes, and when done, drain them and set aside until required. Meanwhile, boil the quinoa in 1 cup water over high heat and then simmer for 15 minutes over low heat until cooked. Prepare the sauce and for this, place a pot over medium heat, add oil, ginger, and garlic, cook for 2 minutes, then stir in turmeric, cook for 1 minute, add tomatoes and cook for 5 minutes. Add remaining ingredients for the sauce, stir until mixed and simmer until ready to serve. Transfer half of the lentils in a food processor, add quinoa and pulse until the mixture resembles sand. Tip the mixture into a bowl, add remaining ingredients for the meatballs and stir until well mixed. Place tofu in a food processor, add

1 tablespoon oil, process until the smooth paste comes together, add to lentil mixture, stir until well mixed and shape the mixture into small balls. Place the balls on a baking sheet, spray with oil and bake for 20 minutes until golden brown. Add balls into the warm sauce, toss until coated, sprinkle with cilantro, and serve.

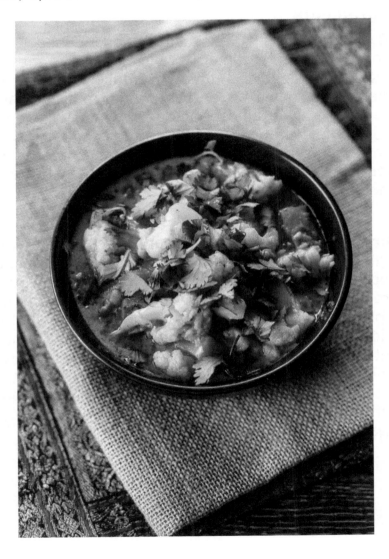

## Stir-Fry Tofu with Mushrooms and Broccoli

Preparation time: 5 minutes

Cooking time: 12 minutes

Servings: 2

### Ingredients:

10 ounces tofu, pressed, drained, cubed 8 ounces broccoli florets, steamed 8 ounces shiitake mushrooms, destemmed, sliced 1 medium shallot, peeled, diced 5 dried red chilies 2 ½ teaspoons minced garlic 2/3 teaspoon salt 2 tablespoons black vinegar, sweetened 2 tablespoons chopped peanuts 2 tablespoons soy sauce 2 tablespoons peanut oil 2 tablespoons water For the Garnish: Sliced scallions as needed Sesame seeds as needed

**Directions:** Take a skillet pan, place it over medium-high heat, add oil and when hot, add some and black pepper, then add tofu cubes and cook for 6 minutes until browned on all sides. When done, transfer tofu cubes to a plate, add garlic and shallots, cook for 2 minutes, then add mushrooms and cook for 3 minutes until tender, add nuts and chilies, and cook for 1 minute. Stir in soy sauce, vinegar and water, add steamed broccoli, toss until well coated, add tofu, toss until mixed, season with salt, and garnish with scallion and sesame seeds. Serve straight away

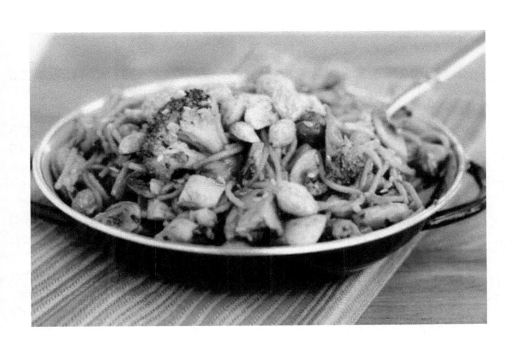

## Roasted Spaghetti Squash with Mushrooms

Preparation time: 10 minutes

Cooking time: 60 minutes

Servings: 4

### Ingredients:

2 pounds spaghetti squash, halved 1 tablespoon unsalted butter 2 tablespoons olive oil ½ of a white onion, peeled, chopped 16 ounces sliced cremini mushrooms 2 teaspoons minced garlic 3 tablespoons sage 2/3 teaspoon salt 1/3 teaspoon ground black pepper 1/8 teaspoon nutmeg ¼ cup grated vegan parmesan cheese

**Directions:** Bake squash on a parchment-lined baking sheet or 50 minutes at 400 degrees F until tender. Meanwhile, take a large skillet pan, place it medium-high heat, add oil and butter and when hot, add onion and cook for 3 minutes until tender. Then add mushrooms, switch heat to medium level, and cook for 7 minutes. Stir in sage and garlic, cook for 4 minutes until mushrooms have turned brown, and then season with black pepper, nutmeg and salt. When squash has roasted, pierce it with a fork, let it cool for 10 minutes, then remove its seeds and scoop the flesh of the squash to a saucepan. Add mushrooms, stir until mixed, season with some more salt, and stir in cheese until incorporated. Serve straight away.

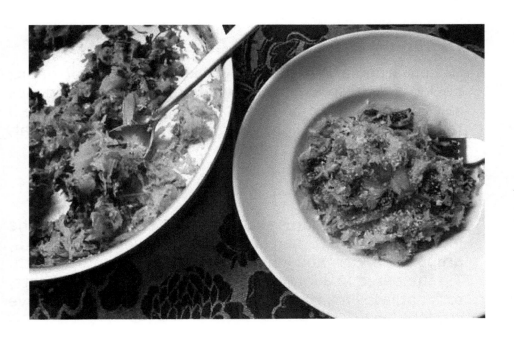

## Avocado Linguine

Preparation time: 10 minutes

Cooking time: 0 minute

Servings: 4

## Ingredients:

½ cup arugula 2 medium avocados 2 cloves of garlic, peeled 1/4 teaspoon ground white pepper 3/4 teaspoons salt 1 teaspoon lemon zest 3 tablespoons lemon juice 3 tablespoons olive oil 8 ounces linguine, whole-wheat, boiled

## Directions:

Prepare the avocado sauce, and for this, place all the ingredients in a food processor, except for pasta, arugula, pepper, and lemon zest and pulse until smooth. Tip the puree in a large bowl, add remaining ingredients, toss until well mixed and taste to adjust seasoning. Serve straight away.

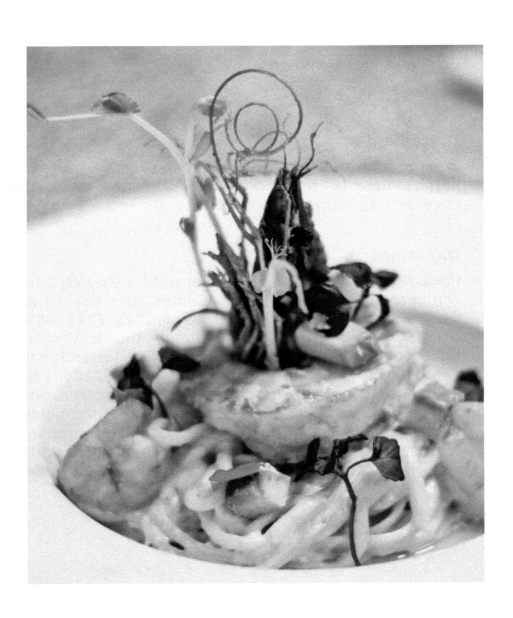

## Scallion Pancakes

Preparation time: 40 minutes

Cooking time: 8 minutes

Servings: 2

## Ingredients:

2 large bunches of green onions, sliced 4 cups all-purpose flour 1/4 teaspoon salt 1/4 cup and 1 tablespoon olive oil 1 1/2 cups chilled water

## Directions:

Place flour in a bowl, stir in water until a smooth dough comes together, knead it for 5 minutes, then cover it with plastic wrap and let it stand for 30 minutes. Then roll the dough into 1/8 thick crust, brush the top with 1 tablespoon oil, season with salt, and scatter with some green onion. Roll the dough into a cigar shape, roll it again into 1/8 inch thick crust and fry it into remaining hot oil for 3 minutes per side until cooked and golden. When done, transfer pancake to a plate lined with paper towels, let it stand for 5 minutes, then cut it into 3 wedges and serve.

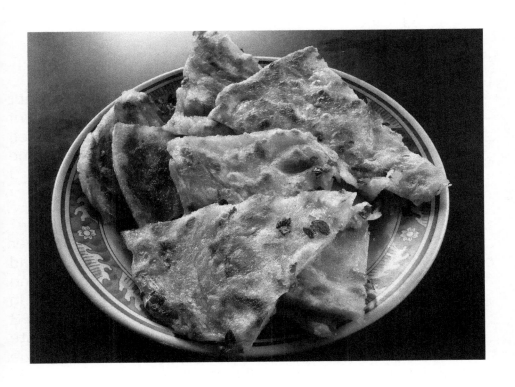

## Mushroom and Broccoli Noodles

Preparation time: 10 minutes

Cooking time: 10 minutes

Servings: 4

### Ingredients:

2 linguine pasta, whole-grain, cooked 8 ounces chestnut mushroom, sliced 4 spring onions, sliced 1 small head of broccoli, cut into florets, steamed ½ teaspoon minced garlic ½ teaspoon red chili flakes 1 tablespoon sesame oil 2 teaspoons hoisin sauce ¼ cup roasted cashew 3 tablespoons stock

**Directions:** Take a large frying pan, place it over medium heat, add oil and when hot, add mushrooms and cook for 2 minutes until golden. Stir in garlic, onion and chili flakes, cook for 1 minute, stir in broccoli and toss in pasta until hot. Drizzle with hoisin sauce and 3 tablespoons of stock, toss until mixed, cook for 1 minute and remove the pan from heat. Top with cashews, drizzle with some more sesame oil and serve.

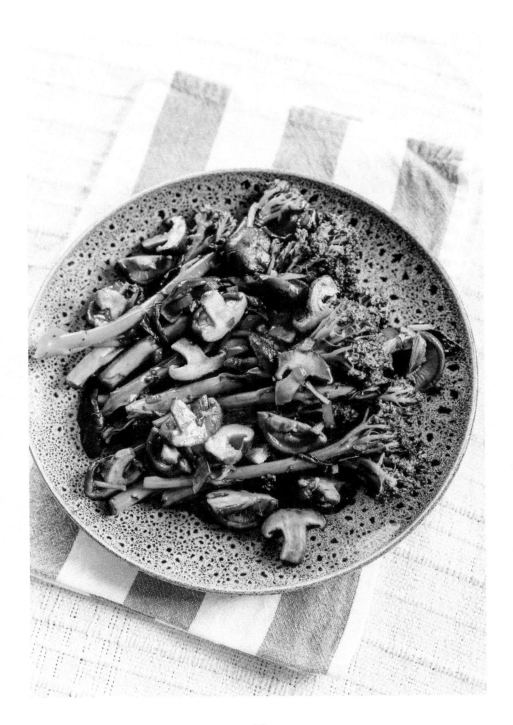

## Pasta with Creamy Greens and Lemon

Preparation time: 5 minutes

Cooking time: 10 minutes

Servings: 4

### Ingredients:

5 ounces broccoli, cut into florets 3.5 ounces frozen soya beans ¼ cup basil leaves 3.5 ounces frozen peas 3.5 ounces mange tout 2/3 teaspoon salt 1/3 teaspoon ground black pepper 1 lemon, juiced, zested 5.3 ounces vegan mascarpone 3 ounces grated vegan parmesan cheese 12 ounces whole-grain pasta, cooked

### Directions:

Cook the pasta in a saucepan, add all the vegetables in the last 3 minutes, and, when done, drain the pasta and vegetables. Return the pasta and vegetables into the pan, add remaining ingredients and stir until well combined. Serve straight away

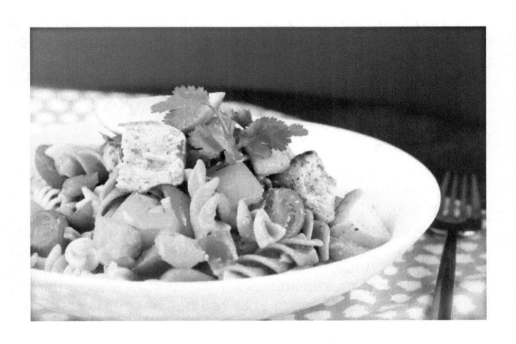

## Dijon Maple Burgers

Serves: 12

Time: 50 Minutes

### Ingredients:

1 Red Bell Pepper 19 Ounces Can Chickpeas, Rinsed & Drained 1 Cup Almonds, Ground 2 Teaspoons Dijon Mustard 1 Teaspoon Oregano ½ Teaspoon Sage 1 Cup Spinach, Fresh 1 – ½ Cups Rolled Oats 1 Clove Garlic, Pressed ½ Lemon, Juiced 2 Teaspoons Maple Syrup, Pure

### Directions:

Get out a baking sheet. Line it with parchment paper. Cut your red pepper in half and then take the seeds out. Place it on your baking sheet, and roast in the oven while you prepare your other ingredients. Process your chickpeas, almonds, mustard and maple syrup together in a food processor. Add in your lemon juice, oregano, sage, garlic and spinach, processing again. Make sure it's combined, but don't puree it. Once your red bell pepper is softened, which should roughly take ten minutes, add this to the processor as well. Add in your oats, mixing well. Form twelve patties, cooking in the oven for a half hour. They should be browned.

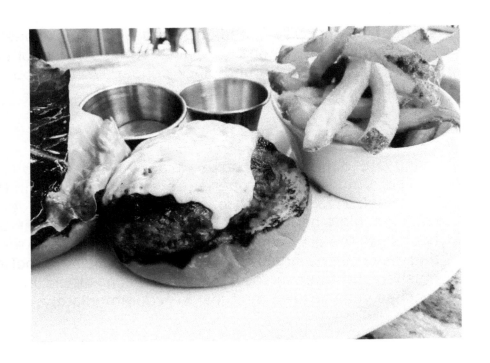

## Flavorful Refried Beans

Servings: 8

Preparation time: 8 hours and 15 minutes

### Ingredients:

3 cups of pinto beans, rinsed 1 small jalapeno pepper, seeded and chopped 1 medium-sized white onion, peeled and sliced 2 tablespoons of minced garlic 5 teaspoons of salt 2 teaspoons of ground black pepper 1/4 teaspoon of ground cumin 9 cups of water

### Directions:

Using a 6-quarts slow cooker, place all the ingredients and stir until it mixes properly. Cover the top, plug in the slow cooker; adjust the cooking time to 6 hours, let it cook on high heat setting and add more water if the beans get too dry. When the beans are done, drain them and reserve the liquid. Mash the beans using a potato masher and pour in the reserved cooking liquid until it reaches your desired mixture. Serve immediately.

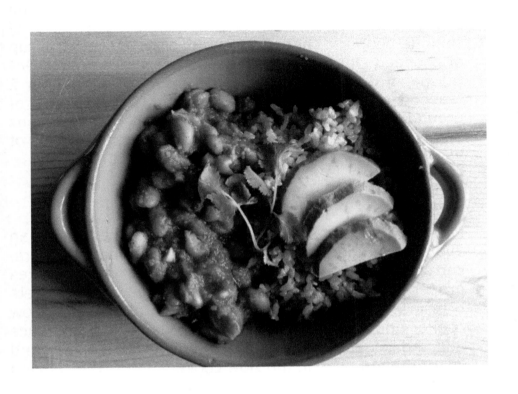

## Spicy Black-Eyed Peas

Servings: 8

Preparation time: 8 hours and 20 minutes

### Ingredients:

32-ounce black-eyed peas, uncooked 1 cup of chopped orange bell pepper 1 cup of chopped celery 8-ounce of chipotle peppers, chopped 1 cup of chopped carrot 1 cup of chopped white onion 1 teaspoon of minced garlic 3/4 teaspoon of salt 1/2 teaspoon of ground black pepper 2 teaspoons of liquid smoke flavoring 2 teaspoons of ground cumin 1 tablespoon of adobo sauce 2 tablespoons of olive oil 1 tablespoon of apple cider vinegar 4 cups of vegetable broth

### Directions:

Place a medium-sized non-stick skillet pan over an average temperature of heat; add the bell peppers, carrot, onion, garlic, oil and vinegar. Stir until it mixes properly and let it cook for 5 to 8 minutes or until it gets translucent. Transfer this mixture to a 6-quarts slow cooker and add the peas, chipotle pepper, adobo sauce and the vegetable broth. Stir until mixes properly and cover the top. Plug in the slow cooker; adjust the cooking time to 8 hours and let it cook on the low heat setting or until peas are soft. Serve right away.

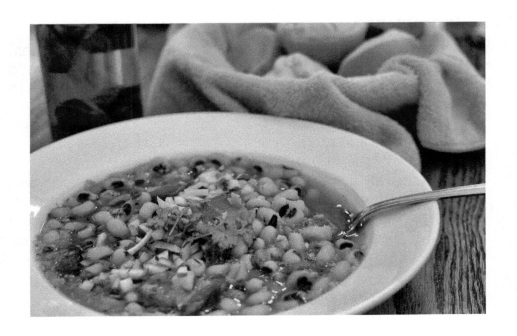

## Tomato Artichoke Soup

Preparation time: 5 minutes

Cooking time: 35 minutes

Servings: 4

## Ingredients:

1 can artichoke hearts, drained 1 can diced tomatoes, undrained 3 cups vegetable broth 1 small onion, chopped 2 cloves garlic, crushed 1 tbsp pesto black pepper, to taste

## Directions:

Combine all ingredients in the slow cooker. Cover and cook on low for 8-10 hours or on high for 4-5 hours. Blend the soup in batches and return it to the slow cooker. Season with salt and pepper to taste and serve.

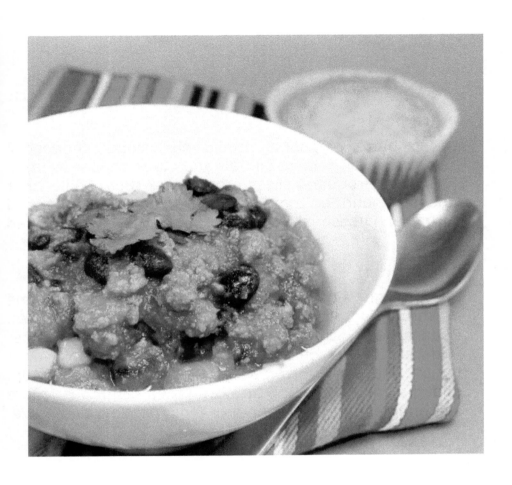

## Mushroom Salad

Preparation time: 10 minutes

Cooking time: 20 minutes

Servings: 2

## Ingredients:

1 tbsp. butter ½ pound cremini mushrooms, chopped 2 tbsp. extra virgin olive oil Salt and black pepper to taste 2 bunches arugula 4 slices prosciutto 1 tbsp. apple cider vinegar 4 sundried tomatoes in oil, drained and chopped Parmesan cheese, shaved Fresh parsley leaves, chopped

## Directions:

Heat a pan with butter and half of the oil. Add the mushrooms, salt, and pepper. Stir-fry for 3 minutes. Reduce heat. Stir again, and cook for 3 minutes more. Add rest of the oil and vinegar. Stir and cook for 1 minute. Place arugula on a platter, add prosciutto on top, add the mushroom mixture, sundried tomatoes, more salt and pepper, parmesan shavings, parsley, and serve.

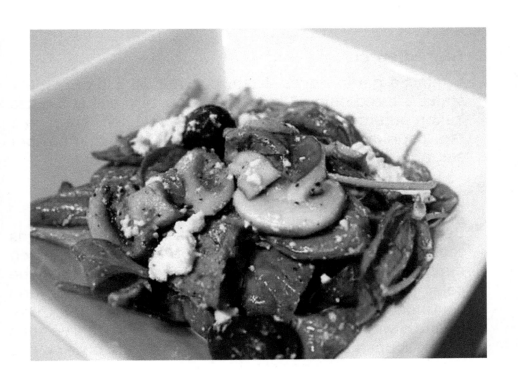

## October Potato Soup

Preparation time: 5 minutes

Cooking time: 20 minutes

3 servings.

## Ingredients:

4 minced garlic cloves 2 tsp. coconut oil 3 diced celery stalks 1 diced onion 2 tsp. yellow mustard seeds 5 diced Yukon potatoes 6 cups vegetable broth 1 tsp. oregano 1 tsp. paprika ½ tsp. cayenne pepper 1 tsp. chili powder salt and pepper to taste

## Directions:

Begin by sautéing the garlic and the mustard seeds together in the oil in a large soup pot. Next, add the onion and sauté the mixture for another five minutes. Add the celery, the broth, the potatoes, and all the spices, and continue to stir. Allow the soup to simmer for thirty minutes without a cover. Next, Position about three cups of the soup in a blender, and puree the soup until you've reached a smooth consistency. Pour this back into the big soup pot, stir, and serve warm. Enjoy.

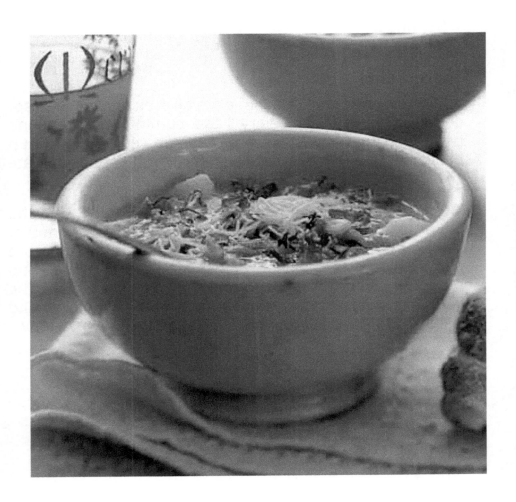

## Lentil Luxury Soup

Preparation time: 5 minutes

Cooking time: 50 minutes

4 Servings.

## Ingredients:

5 minced garlic cloves 1 tsp. olive oil 1 diced onion ½ tsp. coriander 1 cup diced celery 1 tsp. cumin ½ tsp. cayenne pepper 6 cups vegetable broth ¾ cup red lentils ¼ cup black lentils 1 ¼ cup green lentils salt and pepper to taste

**Directions:** Begin by heating the oil, the garlic, and the onion in the bottom of the soup pot for eight minutes. Next, add the celery and the spices. Cook for three more minutes. Add the cooked or canned lentils to the soup pot, next. Pour in the broth and stir well. Next, allow the soup to simmer for forty-five minutes. Stir often. Salt and pepper the soup as you please, and serve warm. Enjoy.

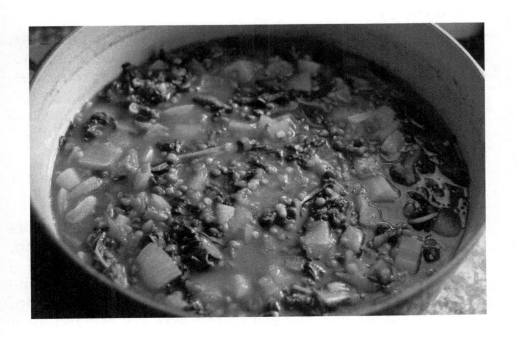

## Exotic Butternut Squash and Chickpea Curry

Servings: 8

Preparation time: 6 hours and 15 minutes

### Ingredients:

1 1/2 cups of shelled peas 1 1/2 cups of chick peas, uncooked and rinsed 2 1/2 cups of diced butternut squash 12 ounce of chopped spinach 2 large tomatoes, diced 1 small white onion, peeled and chopped 1 teaspoon of minced garlic 1 teaspoon of salt 3 tablespoons of curry powder 14-ounce of coconut milk 3 cups of vegetable broth 1/4 cup of chopped cilantro

### Directions:

Using a 6-quarts slow cooker, place all the ingredients into it except for the spinach and peas. Cover the top, plug in the slow cooker; adjust the cooking time to 6 hours and let it cook on the high heat setting or until the chickpeas get tender. 30 minutes to ending your cooking, add the peas and spinach to the slow cooker and let it cook for the remaining 30 minutes. Stir to check the sauce, if the sauce is runny, stir in a mixture of a tablespoon of cornstarch mixed with 2 tablespoons of water. Serve with boiled rice.

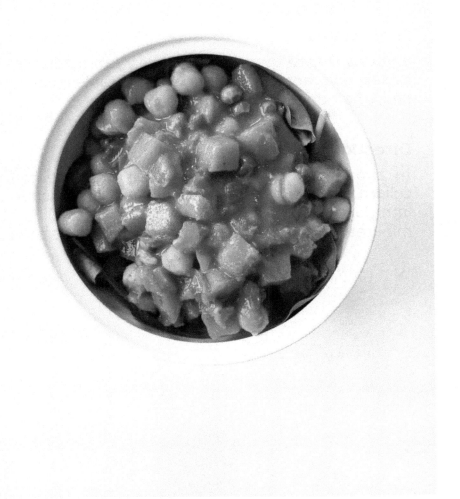

## Collard Greens And Tomatoes

Preparation Time: 10 minutes

Cooking Time: 10 minutes

Servings: 9

### Ingredients

1 pound collard greens ¼ cup cherry tomatoes, halved 1 tablespoon apple cider vinegar 2 tablespoons veggie stock Salt and black pepper to the taste

### Directions:

In a pan that fits your Air Fryer, combine tomatoes, collard greens, vinegar, stock, salt and pepper, stir, introduce in your Air Fryer and cook at 320 ° F for 10 minutes. Divide between plates and serve as a side dish.

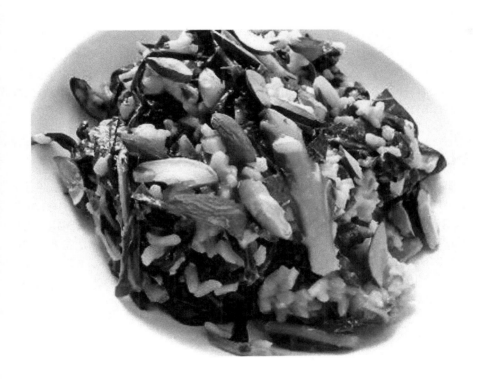

# Creamy Artichoke and Horseradish Soup

Preparation time: 5 minutes

Cooking time: 50 minutes

Servings: 4

## Ingredients:

1 can artichoke hearts, drained 3 cups vegetable broth 1 tbsp vegan horseradish sauce 2 tbsp lemon juice 1 small onion, finely cut 2 cloves garlic, crushed 3 tbsp olive oil 2 tbsp flour 2 tbsp chopped fresh chives plus extra to garnish

## Directions:

Gently sauté the onion and garlic in some olive oil. Add in the flour, whisking constantly, and then add the hot vegetable broth slowly, while still whisking. Cook for about 5 minutes. Blend the artichokes, salt and pepper until smooth. Add the puree to the broth mix, stir well, and then stir in the horseradish sauce and chopped chives. Ladle the soup into bowls and serve.

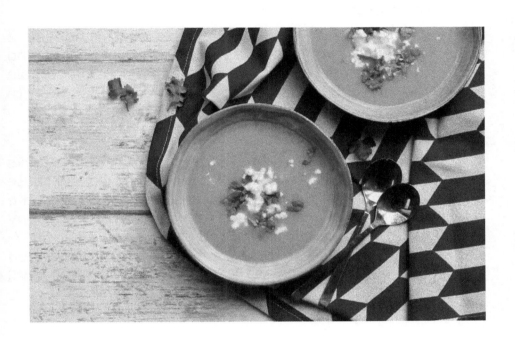

## Celery Root Soup

Preparation time: 5 minutes

Cooking time: 20 minutes

Servings: 4

### Ingredients:

2 leeks (white and light green parts only), chopped 2 garlic cloves, crushed 1 large celery root, peeled and diced 2 potatoes, peeled and diced 4 cups vegetable broth 1 bay leaf 2 tbsp olive oil salt and black pepper, to taste

**Directions:** In a skillet, heat olive oil, then add the leeks and sauté about 3-4 minutes. Add in the garlic and sauté an additional 3-40 seconds. In a slow cooker, add the sautéed leeks and garlic, celeriac, potatoes, broth, bay leaf, salt, and pepper. Cover and cook on low heat for 7-8 hours. Set aside to cool, remove the bay leaf, then process in a blender or with an immersion blender until smooth.

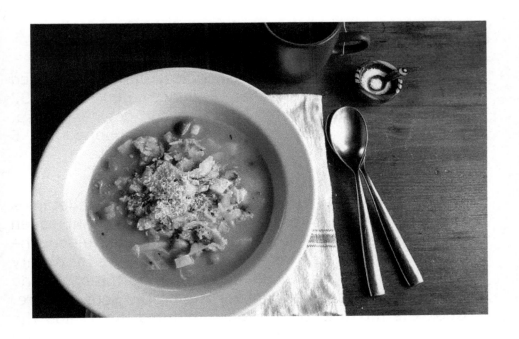

## Quizzical Quinoa Soup

Preparation time: 5 minutes

Cooking time: 20 minutes

6 Servings.

### Ingredients:

1 diced onion 1 tbsp. olive oil 6 diced carrots 3 minced garlic cloves 1 cup quinoa 16 ounces pink beans 32 ounces vegetable broth 2 tsp. curry powder 1 tsp. paprika 2 tsp. curry powder 1/3 cup chopped dill 5 ounces spinach leaves salt and pepper to taste

**Directions:** Begin by heating the oil and the vegetables together in the bottom of a soup pot for about seven minutes. Next, add the vegetable broth, the quinoa, the beans, and all the spices. Simmer this mixture for twenty minutes with the cover on. Next, add the tomatoes and a bit more water to administer the proper soup texture. Cook the mixture for ten more minutes. Next, add the parsley, stir for a few minutes, and then serve the soup instantly. Enjoy!

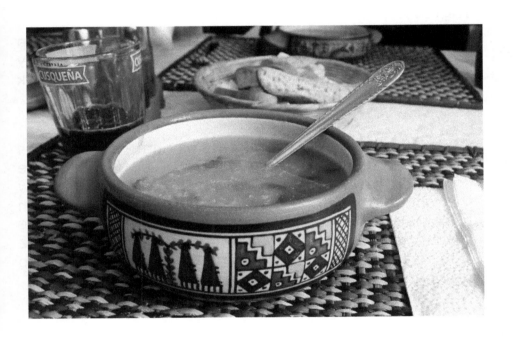

## Barley Country Living Soup

Preparation time: 5 minutes

Cooking time: 30 minutes

8 Servings.

### Ingredients:

2 tbsp. olive oil 32 ounces vegetable broth 1 diced onion 2 diced celery stalks 4 diced carrots 1 ¼ cup pearl barley 12 ounces sliced mushrooms 1 tbsp. basil 2 cups soymilk 1/3 cup minced parsley salt and pepper to taste

**Directions:** Bring by heating the oil and the vegetables together in a soup pot for eight minutes. Next, add the broth, the barley, and the spices to the mixture. Allow the mixture to simmer for fifty minutes with a cover on top. Make sure to stir occasionally. Next, add the soymilk, and season the soup with salt and pepper. Make sure to allow the soup to rest for thirty minutes prior to serving in order to allow it to thicken. Enjoy.

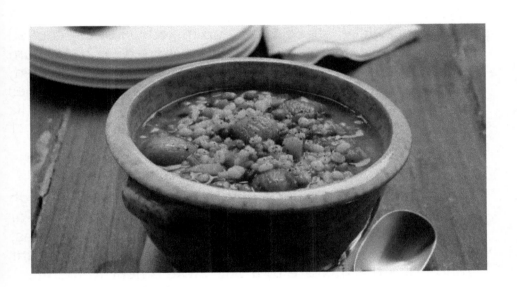

## Lentil and Wild Rice Soup

Preparation time: 10 minutes

Cooking time: 40 minutes

Servings: 4

### Ingredients:

1/2 cup cooked mixed beans 12 ounces cooked lentils 2 stalks of celery, sliced 1 1/2 cup mixed wild rice, cooked 1 large sweet potato, peeled, chopped 1/2 medium butternut, peeled, chopped 4 medium carrots, peeled, sliced 1 medium onion, peeled, diced 10 cherry tomatoes 1/2 red chili, deseeded, diced 1 ½ teaspoon minced garlic 1/2 teaspoon salt 2 teaspoons mixed dried herbs 1 teaspoon coconut oil 2 cups vegetable broth

**Directions:** Take a large pot, place it over medium-high heat, add oil and when it melts, add onion and cook for 5 minutes. Stir in garlic and chili, cook for 3 minutes, then add remaining vegetables, pour in the broth, stir and bring the mixture to a boil. Switch heat to medium-low heat, cook the soup for 20 minutes, then stir in remaining ingredients and continue cooking for 10 minutes until soup has reached to desired thickness. Serve straight away.

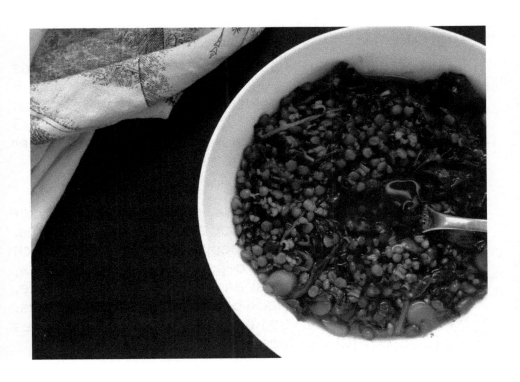

## Black Beans and Cauliflower Rice

Preparation time: 10 minutes

Cooking time: 20 minutes

Servings: 4

### Ingredients:

3 cups cauliflower rice 15.5 ounces cooked black beans 1/2 cup diced red bell pepper 1/2 cup chopped onion 3 tablespoons chopped pickled jalapeno 1 ½ teaspoon minced garlic ¼ teaspoon ground black pepper 1/3 teaspoon sea salt 1/4 teaspoon ground cayenne pepper 2 tablespoons olive oil 1/2 cup diced parsley

**Directions:** Take a large skillet pan, place it over medium heat, add oil and garlic and cook for 2 minutes. Then add onion and bell pepper, season with black pepper, salt, and cayenne pepper, cook for 5 minutes, then stir in jalapeno pepper and top with cauliflower rice. Season with salt and black pepper, cook for 7 minutes, turning halfway, then add beans and cook for 2 minutes until hot. Garnish  with parsley and serve.

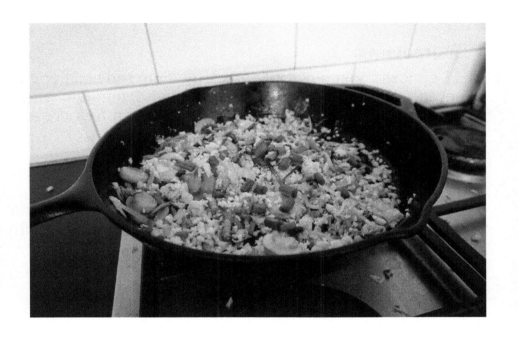

## Black Bean and Quinoa Salad

Preparation time: 10 minutes

Cooking time: 0 minute

Servings: 10

## Ingredients:

15 ounces cooked black beans 1 medium red bell pepper, cored, chopped 1 cup quinoa, cooked 1 medium green bell pepper, cored, chopped 1/2 cup vegan feta cheese, crumbled

## Directions:

Place all the ingredients in a large bowl, except for cheese, and stir until incorporated. Top the salad with cheese and serve straight away.

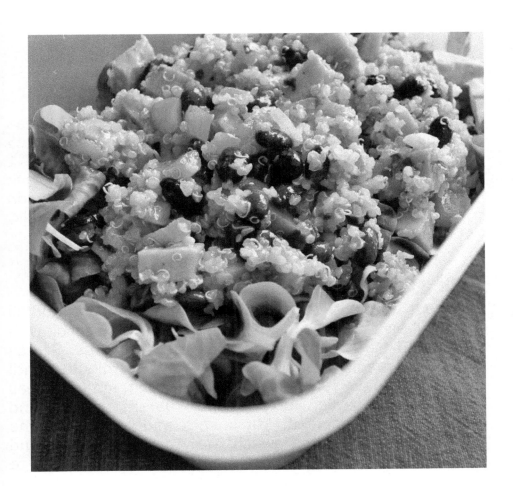

## Coconut Chickpea Curry

Preparation time: 10 minutes

Cooking time: 30 minutes

Servings: 4

### Ingredients:

2 teaspoons coconut flour 16 ounces cooked chickpeas 14 ounces tomatoes, diced 1 large red onion, sliced 1 ½ teaspoon minced garlic ½ teaspoon of sea salt 1 teaspoon curry powder 1/3 teaspoon ground black pepper 1 ½ tablespoons garam masala 1/4 teaspoon cumin 1 small lime, juiced 13.5 ounces coconut milk, unsweetened 2 tablespoons coconut oil

### Directions:

Take a large pot, place it over medium-high heat, add oil and when it melts, add onions and tomatoes, season with salt and black pepper and cook for 5 minutes. Switch heat to medium-low level, cook for 10 minutes until tomatoes have released their liquid, then add chickpeas and stir in garlic, curry powder, garam masala, and cumin until combined. Stir in milk and flour, bring the mixture to boil, then switch heat to medium heat and simmer the curry for 12 minutes until cooked. Taste to adjust seasoning, drizzle with lime juice, and serve

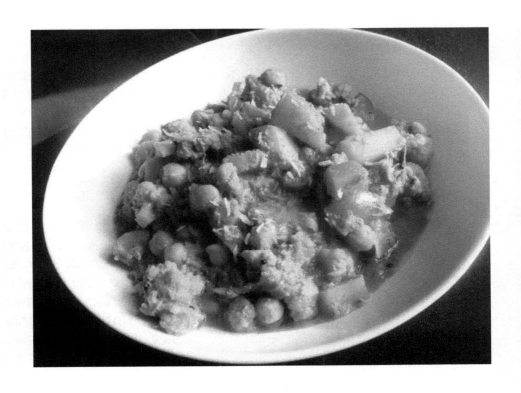

## Zoodles with White Beans

Preparation time: 10 minutes

Cooking time: 20 minutes

Servings: 4

### Ingredients:

15 ounces cooked cannellini beans 2 medium zucchini, spiralized into noodles 3 teaspoons minced garlic 1 cup chopped Roma tomatoes 2/3 teaspoon salt 1/8 teaspoon red pepper flakes 1/4 cup olive oil 1/4 cup chopped parsley 4 ounces whole-grain spaghetti, cooked

### Directions:

Cook the pasta, drain it, transfer it into a bowl, add zucchini noodles and toss until mixed. Take a pot, place it over low heat, add oil, garlic, and red pepper flakes, stir until cook for 5 minutes until garlic is golden brown. Then add all the ingredients, except for parsley and salt, toss until mixed and cook for 5 minutes until thoroughly heated. When done, season with salt, top with parsley and serve.

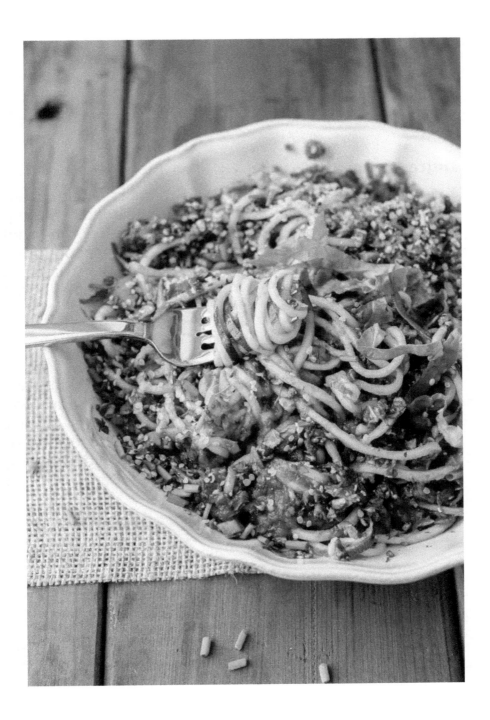

## Pasta with Kidney Bean Sauce

Preparation time: 5 minutes

Cooking time: 15 minutes

Servings: 4

### Ingredients:

12 ounces cooked kidney beans 7 ounces whole-wheat pasta, cooked 1 medium white onion, peeled, diced 1 cup arugula 2 tablespoons tomato paste 1 teaspoon minced garlic ½ teaspoon smoked paprika 1 teaspoon dried oregano ½ teaspoon cayenne pepper 1/3 teaspoon ground black pepper 2/3 teaspoon salt 2 tablespoons balsamic vinegar

### Directions:

Take a large skillet pan, place it over medium-high heat, add onion and garlic, splash with some water and cook for 5 minutes. Then add remaining ingredients, except for pasta and arugula, stir until mixed and cook for 10 minutes until thickened. When done, mash with the fork, top with arugula and serve with pasta. Serve straight away

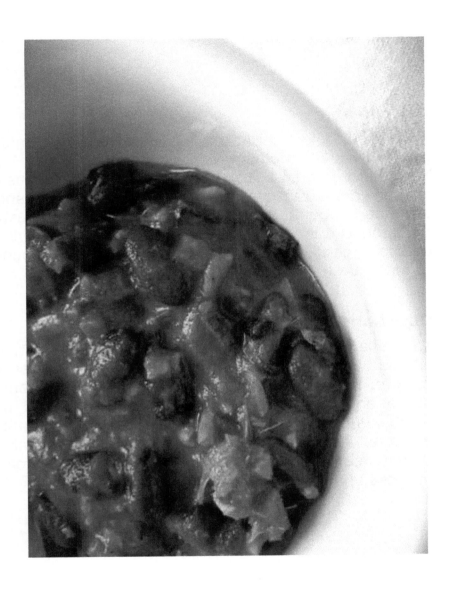

## Chickpea Shakshuka

Preparation time: 5 minutes

Cooking time: 30 minutes

Servings: 6

### Ingredients:

22 ounces cooked chickpeas 1/2 cup diced white onion 5 green olives 1/2 medium red bell pepper, chopped 1 1/2 Tbsp minced garlic 1 Tbsp coconut sugar 2 teaspoons red chili powder 2 teaspoons smoked paprika 1/8 teaspoon cayenne pepper 1 teaspoon salt 3 Tbsp tomato paste 1 tsp ground cumin 1/4 teaspoon ground cinnamon 1/8 teaspoon cardamom 1/8 teaspoon coriander 28-ounces tomato puree 1 Tbsp avocado oil

### Directions:

Take a large skillet pan, place it over medium heat, add oil and when hot, add garlic, onion and bell pepper and cook for 5 minutes until fragrant. Then stir in the tomato puree and tomato paste, stir in all the spices until combined, bring the mixture to simmer, and cook for 3 minutes. Add olives and chickpeas, stir to combine, switch heat to medium-low level and simmer for 20 minutes until cooked. Serve straight away.

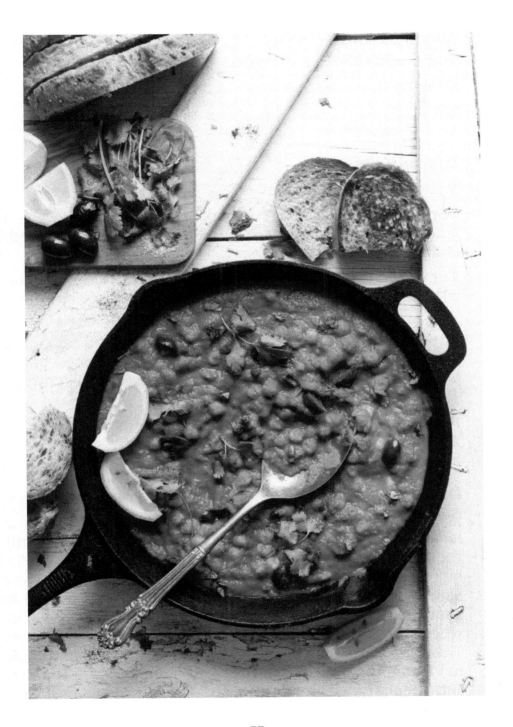

## Avocado Burrito Bowl

Preparation time: 5 minutes

Cooking time: 10 minutes

Servings: 4

### Ingredients:

1 cup brown rice, cooked

**For Marinated Kale:** 1 bunch of kale, chopped ¼ cup lime juice 2 tablespoons olive oil ½ jalapeño, deseeded, chopped ½ teaspoon cumin ¼ teaspoon salt

**For Avocado Salsa:** 1 avocado, pitted, sliced ½ cup cilantro leaves ½ cup salsa verde 2 tablespoons lime juice

**For Seasoned Black Beans:** 1/3 cup chopped red onion 4 cups cooked black beans 1 ½ teaspoon minced garlic ¼ teaspoon cayenne pepper ¼ teaspoon red chili powder 1 tablespoon olive oil

**For Garnish:** 6 Cherry tomatoes, sliced into thin rounds 4 teaspoons hot sauce

### Directions:

Prepare kale and for this, place all its ingredients in a large bowl and toss until combined, set aside until required. Prepare the salsa, and  for this, place all its ingredients in a blender, process until smooth, and set aside until required. Prepare beans and for this, take a saucepan, place it over medium-low heat, add oil and when hot, add onion and garlic and cook for 2 minutes. Then add remaining ingredients, stir until mixed and cook for 7 minutes until beans are heated and tender. Top rice with beans, kale, and salsa, drizzle with hot sauce and serve with tomatoes.

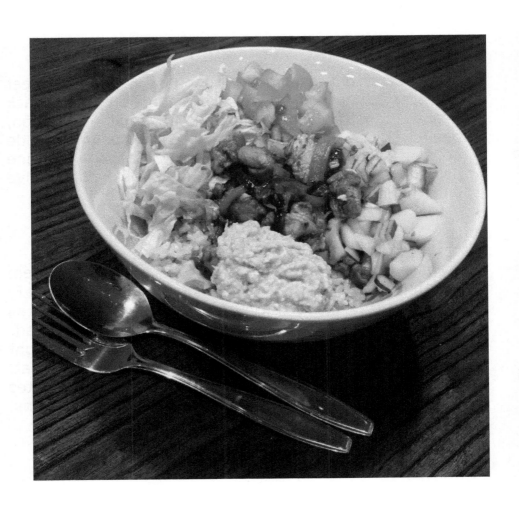

## Sweet Potato and Bean Burgers

Preparation time: 10 minutes

Cooking time: 50 minutes

Servings: 8

### Ingredients:

1 cup oats, old-fashioned, ground 1 ½ pounds sweet potatoes 1 cup cooked millet 15 ounces cooked black beans ½ cup cilantro, chopped ½ small red onion, peeled, diced ½ teaspoon salt 1 teaspoon chipotle powder 2 teaspoons cumin powder ½ teaspoon cayenne powder 1 teaspoon red chili powder 2 tablespoons olive oil 8 hamburger buns, whole-wheat, toasted

### Directions:

Prepare sweet potatoes, and for this, slice them lengthwise and roast for 40 minutes at 400 degrees F, cut-side up. Prepare the burgers and for this, place all the ingredients in the bowl, except for oil and buns, stir until combined, and then shape the mixture into eight patties. Take a skillet pan, place it over medium heat, add oil and when hot, add patties and cook for 4 minutes per side until browned. Sandwich patties between buns, and serve.

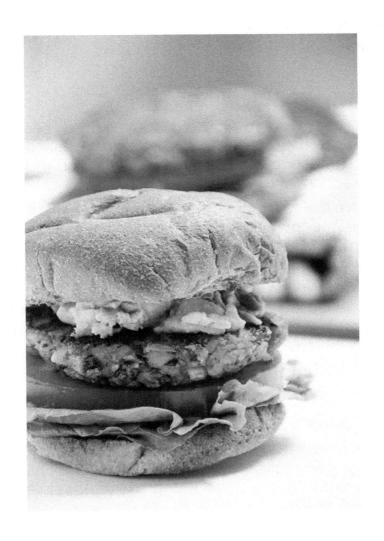

## Burrito-Stuffed Sweet Potatoes

Preparation time: 10 minutes

Cooking time: 45 minutes

Servings: 4

### Ingredients:

**For Sweet Potatoes:** 1 cup cooked black beans 4 small sweet potatoes ½ cup of brown rice ½ teaspoon minced garlic 1 teaspoon tomato paste 1 teaspoon ground cumin ¼ teaspoon salt ½ teaspoon olive oil 1 ¼ cup water

**For the Salsa:** 1 cup cherry tomatoes, halved 1 medium red bell pepper, deseeded, chopped ¾ cup chopped red onion 2 tablespoon chopped cilantro leaves ½ teaspoon salt ¼ teaspoon ground black pepper 1 ½ teaspoon olive oil 1 tablespoon lime juice

**For the Guacamole:**  1 medium avocado, pitted, peeled ½ teaspoon minced garlic 2 tablespoons chopped cilantro leaves ¼ teaspoon salt 1 tablespoon lime juice

**For Serving:** Shredded cabbage as needed

### Directions:

Prepare sweet potatoes and for this, place them in a baking dish, prick them with a fork and bake for 45 minutes at 400 degrees F until very tender. Meanwhile, place a medium saucepan over medium heat, add rice and beans, stir in salt, oil, and tomatoes paste, pour in water and bring the mixture to boil. Switch heat to medium-low level, simmer for 40 minutes until all the liquid has absorbed and set aside until required. Prepare the salsa and for this, place all its ingredients in a bowl and stir until combined, set aside until required. Prepare the guacamole and for this, place the avocado in a bowl, mash well, then add remaining ingredients, stir until combined, and set aside until required. When sweet potatoes are baked, cut them along the top, pull back the skin, then split and top with rice and beans mixture. Top with salsa and guacamole and cabbage and serve.

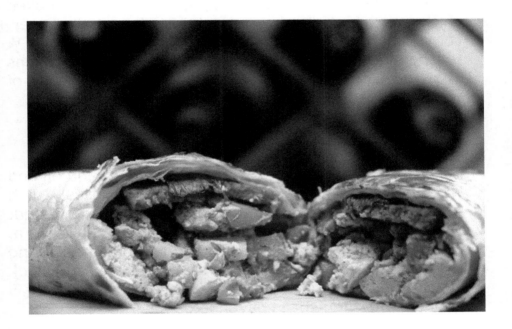

## Sweet Potato, Kale and Chickpea Soup

Preparation time: 10 minutes

Cooking time: 50 minutes

Servings: 6

### Ingredients:

3 cups cooked farro 3 cups chopped kale 1 ½ cups cooked chickpeas 3 cups diced sweet potatoes 1 red bell pepper, cored, chopped 1 large white onion, peeled, chopped ¼ teaspoon salt ¼ teaspoon cayenne pepper 2 tablespoons Thai red curry paste 2 tablespoons olive oil 2 cups of water 4 cups vegetable broth

### Directions:

Take a large pot, place it over medium heat, add oil and when hot, add onion, potato and bell pepper, season with salt, and cook for 5 minutes until onions have softened. Stir in curry paste, cook for 1 minute, then stir in farro, pour in water and broth, and stir until combined. Bring the mixture to boil, switch heat to the low level and cook for 35 minutes. Stir in kale and chickpeas, cook for 5 minutes and then stir in cayenne pepper.

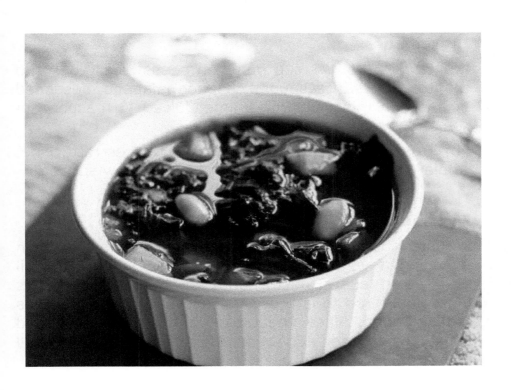

## Pesto with Squash Ribbons and Fettuccine

Preparation time: 10 minutes

Cooking time: 0 minute

Servings: 4

### Ingredients:

**For the Pesto** 1/3 cup pumpkin seeds, toasted 1 cup cilantro leaves 2 teaspoons chopped jalapeño, deseeded 1 teaspoon minced garlic 1 lime, juiced ½ teaspoon of sea salt ⅓ cup olive oil

**For Pasta and Squash Ribbons** 8 ounces fettuccine, whole-grain, cooked 2 small zucchini 1 yellow squash

### Directions:

Prepare ribbons, and for this, slice zucchini and squash by using a vegetable peeler and then set aside until required. Prepare pesto, and for this, place all its ingredients in a food processor and pulse for 2 minutes until blended. Place vegetable ribbons in a bowl, add cooked pasta, then add prepared pesto and toss until well coated. Serve straight away.

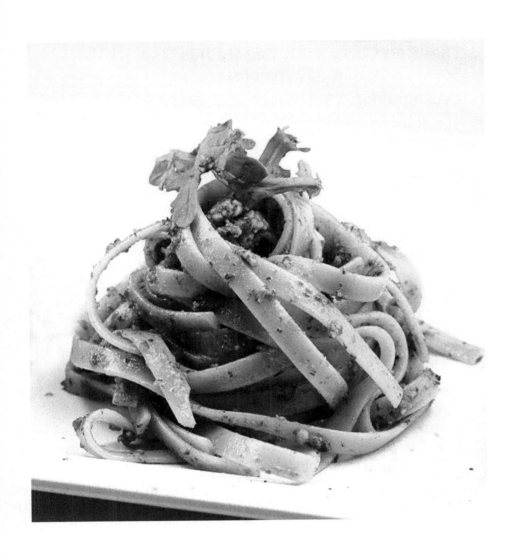

## Thai Red Curry with Vegetables

Preparation time: 10 minutes

Cooking time: 25 minutes

Servings: 4

### Ingredients:

1 ¼ cups brown rice, cooked 1 cup sliced carrots 1 medium red bell pepper, cored, sliced into strips 1 green bell pepper, cored, sliced into strips 1 ½ cups sliced kale 1 teaspoon minced garlic 1 cup chopped white onion 1 tablespoon grated ginger 1/8 teaspoon salt 2 tablespoons Thai red curry paste 1 ½ teaspoon coconut sugar 1 tablespoon olive oil 1 tablespoon soy sauce 2 teaspoons lime juice 14 ounces of coconut milk ½ cup of water ¼ cup chopped cilantro

### Directions:

Prepare the curry and for this, take a large skillet pan, place it over medium heat, add oil and when hot, add onion, season with salt, and cook for 5 minutes. Stir in ginger and garlic, cook for 1 minute until fragrant, then add carrot and bell pepper and cook for 5 minutes. Stir in curry paste, cook for 2 minutes, then add kale, stir in sugar, pour in coconut milk, stir until combined and bring the mixture to simmer. Switch heat to the low level, simmer for 10 minutes until vegetables are tender, and then stir in soy sauce and lime juice. Garnish with cilantro and serve with brown rice.

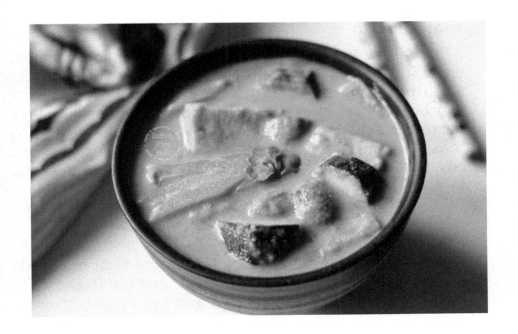

## Thai Green Curry with Spring Vegetables

Preparation time: 10 minutes

Cooking time: 35 minutes

Servings: 4

### Ingredients:

2 cups sliced asparagus 1 small white onion, peeled, diced 2 cups baby spinach, chopped 1 cup sliced carrots 1 teaspoon minced garlic 1 tablespoon chopped ginger 1 cup brown rice, cooked 2 tablespoons Thai green curry paste 1 ½ teaspoon coconut sugar 1/8 teaspoon salt 1 ½ teaspoon lime juice 2 teaspoons olive oil 1 ½ teaspoons soy sauce 14 ounces coconut milk, unsweetened ½ cup of water

### Directions:

Take a large skillet pan, place it over medium heat, add oil and when hot, add ginger, onion, and garlic and cook for 5 minutes. Then add carrots and asparagus, cook for 3 minutes, stir in curry paste and continue cooking for 2 minutes. Pour in milk and water, stir in sugar and bring the curry to simmer. Switch heat to the low level, simmer for 10 minutes until cooked, then stir in spinach and cook for 30 seconds until spinach leaves wilt. When done, remove the pan from heat, stir in lime juice and soy sauce, taste to adjust seasoning and garnish with cilantro. Serve curry with boiled rice.

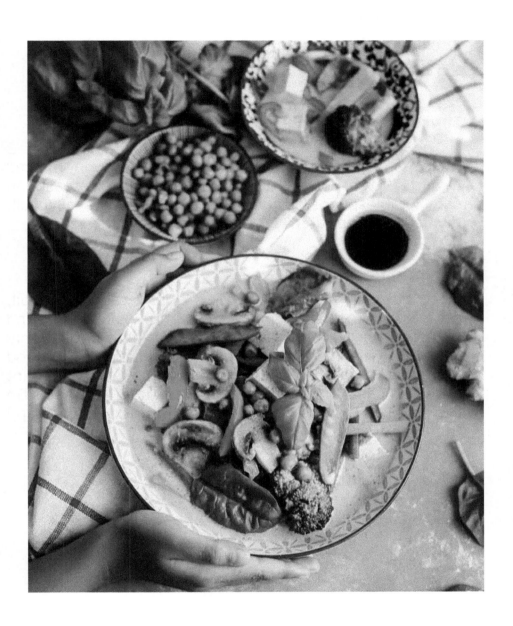

## Zucchanoush

Preparation time: 10 minutes

Cooking time: 10 minutes

Servings: 7

### Ingredients:

1 pound small zucchini, quartered lengthwise 3 tablespoons mint leaves, divided ½ teaspoon minced garlic 1/3 teaspoon ground black pepper 2/3 teaspoon salt 2 tablespoons lemon juice 3 tablespoons olive oil, divided 1/4 cup tahini 1 tablespoon pine nuts, toasted

### Directions:

Place zucchini pieces in a bowl, add 1 tablespoon oil, season with ½ teaspoon salt, toss until well coated, and then grill for 10 minutes over medium heat until evenly charred. Then transfer grilled zucchini to a food processor, add remaining ingredients, except for mint and nuts, and process for 2 minutes until blended. Tip the mixture in a bowl, garnish with mint and nuts and then serve.

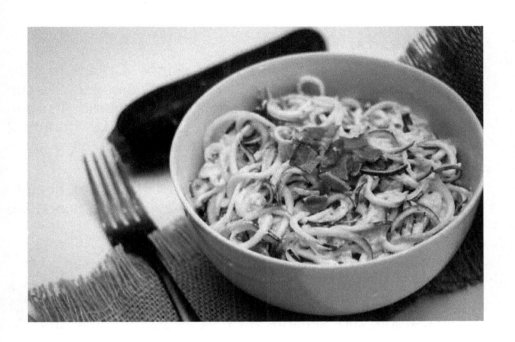

## Mushroom and Quinoa Burger

Preparation time: 15 minutes

Cooking time: 40 minutes

Servings: 5

### Ingredients:

**For the Burgers:** 1 cup cooked quinoa 4 medium caps of Portobello mushroom, gills removed, chopped 1/4 cup chopped red onion ½ teaspoon minced garlic 3 green onions, chopped 1/2 cup cornstarch 1/2 cup walnuts 2 teaspoons rice wine vinegar 2 tablespoons olive oil 5 whole-grain burger buns

**For Toppings:** Sprouts as needed Lettuce as needed Sliced tomatoes as needed Vegan mayonnaise as needed

### Directions:

Prepare the burgers and for this, place mushrooms in a baking dish, add garlic and nuts, drizzle with 1 tablespoon oil, season with ¾ teaspoon salt and ¼ teaspoon black pepper, and then bake for 20 minutes until tender. Then transfer the mushroom mixture in a food processor, add remaining ingredients for a burger, except for buns, stir until well mixed and then shape the mixture into five patties. Fry the patties in batches for 5 minutes until browned and then bake for 10 minutes at 375 degrees F until thoroughly cooked. Sandwich patties in burger buns, top with mayonnaise, sprouts, lettuce and tomatoes, and then serve.

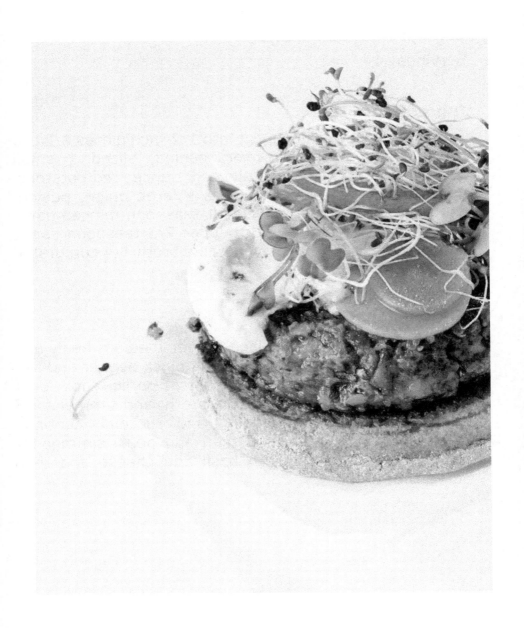

## Summer Minestrone

Preparation time: 5 minutes

Cooking time: 15 minutes

Servings: 4

## Ingredients:

1 medium yellow squash, cut into 1/2-inch pieces 1/2 cup frozen peas 1 small carrot, peeled, sliced 1 small zucchini, cut into 1/2-inch pieces 8 ounces red potatoes, peeled, cut into 1/2-inch pieces 1 large onion, peeled, chopped 1 tablespoon olive oil 1 teaspoon minced garlic 1/3 teaspoon ground black pepper 2/3 teaspoon salt 1 cup chopped basil 4 cups vegetable broth 1/4 cup grated vegan parmesan cheese

## Directions:

Take a large saucepan, place it over medium heat, add oil and when hot, add onion, stir in black pepper and salt and cook for 8 minutes. Then stir in garlic, cook for 1 minute, stir in potatoes, pour in broth and simmer for 5 minutes. Add carrot, squash, and zucchini, continue simmer for 3 minutes, and then add peas, simmer for another 3 minutes. Stir in basil and cheese and then serve with bread

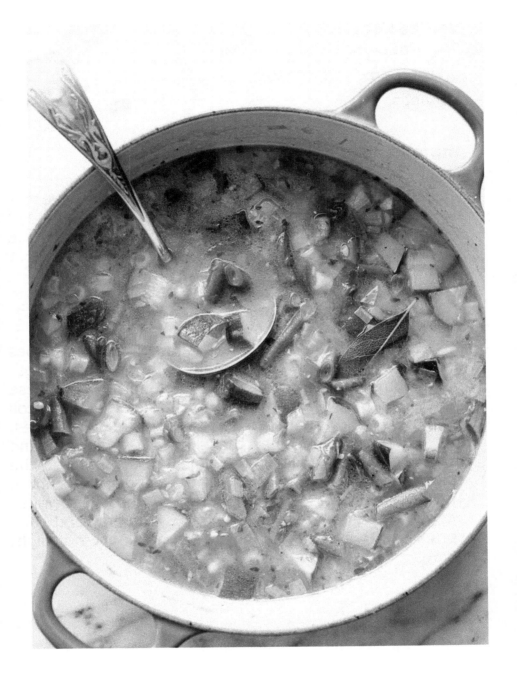

## Veggie Kabobs

Preparation time: 10 minutes

Cooking time: 10 minutes

Servings: 10

### Ingredients:

8 ounces button mushrooms, halved 2 pounds summer squash, peeled, 1-inch cubed 12 ounces small broccoli florets 2 cups grape tomatoes 1 teaspoon salt 1/2 teaspoon smoked paprika 1 teaspoon ground cumin 6 tablespoons olive oil 1/2 teaspoon ground coriander 1 lime, juiced

### Directions:

Toss broccoli florets with 1 tablespoon oil, toss tomatoes and squash pieces with 2 tablespoons oil, then toss mushrooms with 1 tablespoon oil and thread these vegetables onto skewers. Grill mushrooms and broccoli for 7 to 10 minutes, squash and tomatoes and 8 minutes, and when done, transfer the skewers to a plate and drizzle with lime juice and remaining oil. Prepared the spice mix and for this, stir together salt, paprika, cumin, and coriander, sprinkle half of the mixture over grilled veggies, cover them with foil for 5 minutes, and then sprinkle with the remaining spice mix. Serve straight away.

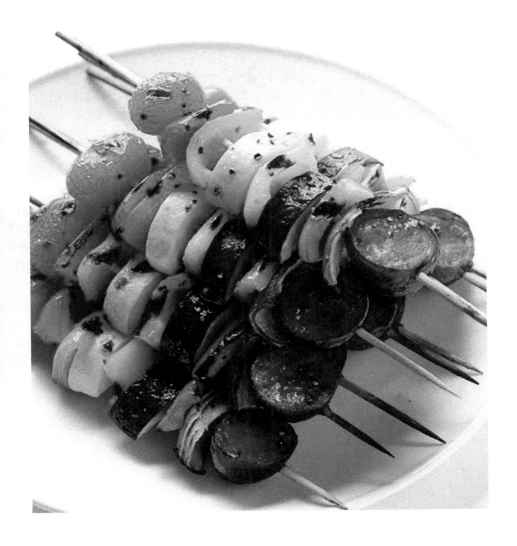

# Linguine with Wild Mushrooms

Preparation time: 5 minutes

Cooking time: 3 minutes

Servings: 4

## Ingredients:

12 ounces mixed mushrooms, sliced 2 green onions, sliced 1 ½ teaspoon minced garlic 1 pound whole-grain linguine pasta, cooked 1/4 cup nutritional yeast ½ teaspoon salt ¾ teaspoon ground black pepper 6 tablespoons olive oil ¾ cup vegetable stock, hot

## Directions:

Take a skillet pan, place it over medium-high heat, add garlic and mushroom and cook for 5 minutes until tender. Transfer the vegetables to a pot, add pasta and remaining ingredients, except for green onions, toss until combined and cook for 3 minutes until hot. Garnish with green onions and serve.

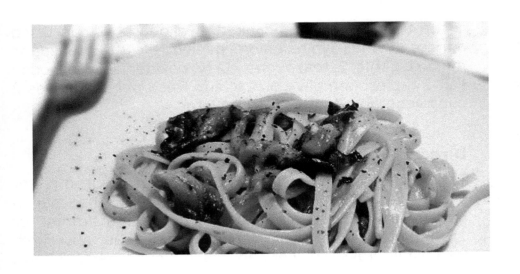

# Pilaf with Garbanzos and Dried Apricots

Preparation time: 10 minutes

Cooking time: 15 minutes

Servings: 4

## Ingredients:

1 cup bulgur 6 ounces cooked chickpeas 1/2 cup Dried apricot 1 small white onion, peeled, diced ½ teaspoon minced garlic 2 teaspoons curry powder 1/2 teaspoon salt 1 tablespoon olive oil 1/4 cup fresh parsley leaves 2 cups vegetable broth 3/4 cup water

## Directions:

Take a saucepan, place it over high heat, pour in water and 1 ½ cup broth, and bring it to a boil. Then stir in bulgur, switch heat to medium-low level and simmer for 15 minutes until most of the liquid has absorbed. Meanwhile, take a skillet pan, place it over medium heat, add oil and when hot, add onion, cook for 10 minutes, then stir in garlic and curry powder and cook for another minute. Then add apricots, beans, and salt, pour in remaining broth and bring the mixture to boiling. Remove pan from heat, fluff the bulgur with a fork, add to the onion-apricot mixture and stir until mixed. Garnish with parsley and serve.

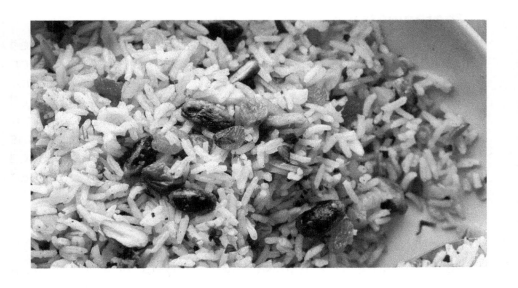

# Kung Pao Brussels Sprouts

Preparation time: 10 minutes

Cooking time: 25 minutes

Servings: 1

## Ingredients:

2 pounds Brussels sprouts, halved 1 teaspoon minced garlic ¾ teaspoon ground black pepper 1 tablespoon cornstarch 1 ½ teaspoon salt 1 tablespoon brown sugar 1/8 teaspoon red pepper flakes 1 tablespoon sesame oil 2 tablespoons olive oil 2 teaspoons apple cider vinegar 1/2 cup soy sauce 1 tablespoon hoisin sauce 2 teaspoons garlic chili sauce 1/2 cup water Sesame seeds as needed for garnish Green onions as needed for garnish Chopped roasted peanuts as needed for garnish

## Directions:

Place sprouts on a baking sheet, drizzle with oil, season with salt and black pepper, and then bake for 20 minutes at 425 degrees F until crispy and tender. Meanwhile, take a skillet pan, place it over medium heat, add oil and when hot, add garlic and cook for 1 minute until fragrant. Then stir in cornstarch and remaining ingredients, except for garnishing ingredients and simmer for 3 minutes, set aside until required. When Brussel sprouts have roasted, add them to the sauce, toss until mixed and broil for 5 minutes until glazed. When done, garnish with nuts, sesame seeds, and green onions and then serve.

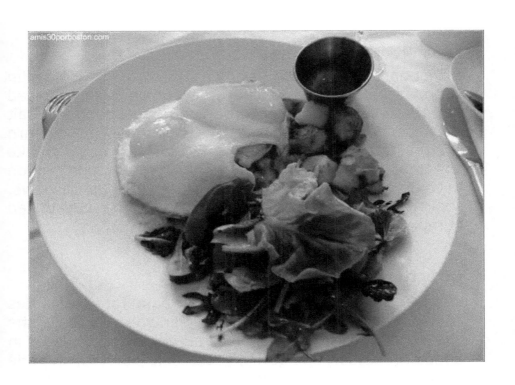

## Stuffed Sweet Potato

Preparation time: 10 minutes

Cooking time: 45 minutes

Servings: 4

### Ingredients:

4.5 pounds sweet potatoes 1/3 cup corn kernels 1 cup chopped kale 1/4 cup diced green onion 3/4 cup diced tomato ½ teaspoon minced garlic 1/2 teaspoon sea salt 1/2 teaspoon chipotle flakes 1/2 teaspoon Dijon mustard 1/2 teaspoon smoked paprika 1/2 teaspoon liquid smoke 1/4 teaspoon ground turmeric 1/2 tablespoon lemon juice 3 tablespoons nutritional yeast 1/3 cup cashews, soaked, drained 1 1/2 cup pasta, cooked 1 cup baked pumpkin puree 1/2 cup vegetable broth

### Directions:

Wrap each potato in a foil and then bake for 45 minutes at 375 degrees F until tender. Meanwhile, prepare the cheese sauce and for this, place pumpkin and cashews in a food processor, add garlic, yeast, salt, paprika, chipotle flakes, liquid smoke, turmeric, mustard, and lemon juice, pour in broth and puree until smooth. Take a pot, place it over medium-low heat, add prepared sauce, then add remaining ingredients, toss until coated, and cook for 5 minutes until kale has wilted. Season the mixture with salt and black pepper, then switch heat to the low level and cook until sweet potatoes have roasted. When sweet potatoes are roasted, let them stand for 10  minutes, then unwrap them, split them by slicing down the center and spoon prepared sauce generously in the center. Serve straight away.

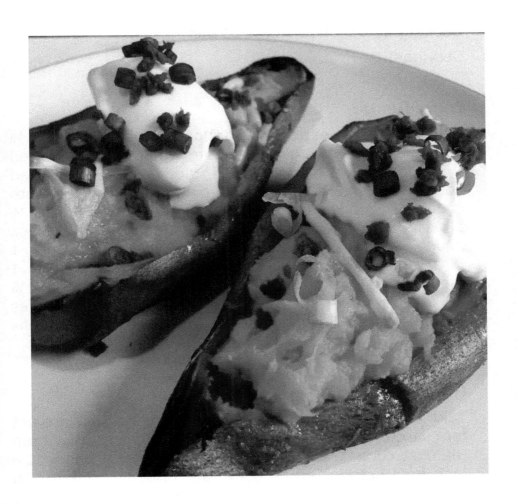

## Tofu Tikka Masala

Preparation time: 10 minutes

Cooking time: 4 hours and 10 minutes

Servings: 4

### Ingredients:

16 ounces tofu, extra-firm, drained, ½ inch cubed 1 ½ teaspoon minced garlic 2 medium carrots, peeled sliced 1 medium white onion, peeled, diced 1 1/2 cups diced potatoes 1 medium red bell pepper, cored, cut into chunks ¾ cup frozen peas 2 cups cauliflower florets ½ tablespoon grated ginger ¼ teaspoon ground black pepper ½ teaspoon salt ½ teaspoon ground turmeric 1 ½ teaspoons cumin ¼ teaspoon cayenne pepper 1 tablespoon garam masala 1 teaspoon coriander ¼ teaspoon paprika ½ tablespoon maple syrup 15 ounces tomato sauce 15 ounces of coconut milk 2 tablespoons chopped cilantro

### Directions:

Take a slow cooker, place all the ingredients in it, except for cilantro and peas, and stir until combined. Switch on the slow cooker, shut with lid, and cook for 4 hours at a high heat setting. When done, stir in peas, cook for 10 minutes, uncovering the cooker, and, when done, serve with cooked brown rice.

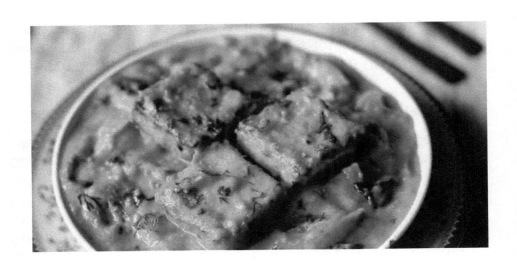

# Buffalo Cauliflower Tacos

Preparation time: 10 minutes

Cooking time: 20 minutes

Servings: 4

## Ingredients:

**For the Cauliflower:** 1/2 head cauliflower, cut into florets 1 teaspoon garlic powder ¼ teaspoon ground black pepper 1 teaspoon red chili powder 4 teaspoons olive oil 3/4 cup buffalo sauce

**For The Tacos:** 1 medium head of romaine lettuce, chopped 8 flour tortillas 1 medium avocado, pitted, diced Vegan ranch as needed Chopped cilantro as needed

## Directions:

Place cauliflower florets in a bowl, add garlic powder, black pepper,  red chili powder, olive oil, and ¼ cup buffalo sauce and toss until combined. Spread cauliflower florets on a baking sheet in a single layer and cook for 20 minutes until roasted, flipping halfway. When done, transfer cauliflower in a large bowl, then heat remaining buffalo sauce, add to cauliflower florets and toss until combined. Assemble tacos and for this, top tortilla with cauliflower, lettuce, and avocado, drizzle with ranch dressing and then top with green onions. Serve straight away.

Lightning Source UK Ltd.
Milton Keynes UK
UKHW020809250521
384334UK00001B/100